Shom

KU-377-336

HERBAL TEAS

Herbal Teas, apart from being much better for you than the popular Indian or China teas, make delicious drinks and can 'dispel all manner of discomforts'. The author – lifelong naturalist, broadcaster and contributor to *The Times* – describes over a hundred herbs and gives instructions for making and using the teas.

By the same author

HERBS AND FRUIT FOR SLIMMERS
HERBS AND FRUIT FOR VITAMINS
HERBS FOR FIRST-AID AND MINOR AILMENTS
HERBS TO HELP YOU SLEEP
HERBS FOR ACIDITY AND GASTRIC ULCERS
FREE FOR ALL: Weeds and Wild Plants as a
    Source of Food

HERBAL TEAS
for Health and Healing

by

CERES

Illustrated by Alison Ross

THORSONS PUBLISHERS LIMITED
Wellingborough, Northamptonshire

First published September 1976
Second Impression October 1976
Third Impression August 1977

© CERES ESPLAN 1976

This book is sold subject to the condition that it shall not, by way of trade or otherwise, be lent, hired out, or otherwise circulated without the publisher's prior consent in any form of binding or cover other than that in which it is published and without a similar condition including this condition being imposed on the subsequent purchaser.

ISBN 0 7225 0339 3

Filmset by Specialised Offset Services Ltd., Liverpool
Printed and bound in Great Britain by
Weatherby Woolnough, Wellingborough,
Northamptonshire

CONTENTS

INTRODUCTION

It was the Romans who boasted that they could do without doctors because of their great knowledge of medicinal herbs. They brought many with them, including Sage, Thyme, Rosemary, Southernwood, Chives, Onion, Borage, Parsley, Rue, and Fennel, so they certainly enhanced our native repertory.

Unfortunately, since their day, our confidence in the virtues of herbs has lessened a little. Possibly some of us are blinded by the glamour of modern medical science, but no one who has enough interest to study the traditional attributes of plants ought to dismiss them without trying some of their old, simple, curative and harmless effects for themselves.

Qualified medical herbalists are available in many places to offer professional advice and they can guide their patients towards the sensible use of correct herbs for various illnesses. But, for minor ailments, there is normally no reason why the many plentiful harmless herbs which can 'dispel all manner of discomforts' should not be tried out in the home.

Some of the herbal teas described in this book make delicious drinks, which once tasted are never neglected again, and some are so efficacious in helping individuals over commonplace little maladies, that they too are in constant use.

There is no description of tea, which is obviously the best known, apart from beer perhaps, of all herbal drinks. This is because I believe that Indian and China Tea are to be avoided as they do not do anyone much good. There are plenty of less addictive substitutes with tea's stimulant properties.

It seems now extraordinary that the discovery of the teaplant (*Camellia sinensis*) by tribesmen in Southern China so many thousands of years ago should have played such a big part in our lives.

No one could deny the romance of the clippers racing over the oceans to bring their tea cargoes back, nor indeed other less fast journeys with the same object – overland by caravans of pack-animals – but it is nevertheless surprising that the profitable enterprise is still so popular. The world produces over a million tons of dried tea a year and Britain is its largest importer! It is sad that tea, 'tay', 'char', or 'the old lady's favourite', should hold top place in the popularity stakes among herbal teas.

It is sad because it is not wholly a beneficial drink. The stimulant, 'theine', which tea contains is an alkaline similar to the dubious 'caffeine', the imbibing of which is habit-forming. The longer brewed tea is kept, too, the stronger its 'tannin' content.

'Tannin' is an astringent and bad for the digestion because it is drying to the lining of the stomach and therefore hindering to the production of essential digestive juices.

There are, of course, plenty of available references to the benefits of drinking herbal teas, or *tisanes*, in the different herbals of most countries. Some are difficult to find, not having been translated into English, others are complicated to read, so this book is an introduction to the great variety of plants that can be used, often free, as many are weeds or even common garden plants, instead of tea as we know it.

Herbal teas have their own virtues. Some are slightly stimulating, like the drinks or infusions made from the 'cordial' plants. Others are tonics or refreshing alteratives, which, given time, can put an 'out of gear' system back to complete health. Many 'lift' melancholy and depression. Some are soothing and induce quiet sleep, or act as daytime tranquillizers, and others alleviate pain, or clear the skin, or act as mild digestives.

Certainly a few herbs for tea-making have to be imported: the delicious Jasmine tea is compounded from two species of this fragrant plant which grows in China, and the tough and carefully prepared little leaves of one of the most valuable teaplants in the world – Maté – was originally only enjoyed in South America. The American Indians discovered the invaluable 'Bonesets' or species of *Eupatoria*, which have vast medical possibilities.

The Indians are known to have taught the settlers about many herbal teas and we have all become indebted to their immense knowledge of plants. It is to be hoped that the settlers, in their turn, passed on some of our European and English knowledge of the herbs that they took with them on their hazardous voyages to the new lands.

History recalls that in the 'tea-less' period in seventeenth-century America, when such a stand was taken in protest against the import clause in the Revenue Act, many women discovered herbal teas which were new to them. 'Liberty Tea', made from the leaves of *Ceanothus*, was one and 'Oswego Tea', from the red flowers of Bergamot, another.

They also tried, or so it is said, Raspberry-leaf tea then. This is a traditional drink for the last few weeks in pregnancy when, if it is taken regularly, it does much to lessen the duration and pain of childbirth, but even the most ardent herbal tea-drinker could not call it at all pleasant.

Raspberry-leaf tea, and others with bland or even slightly unpleasant tastes, if prescribed to help to overcome difficult periods, can be made palateable with the addition of a little honey, or a slice of lemon or a curl of orange peel. None should be abandoned without a fair trial, for it is astonishing how quickly tastes can be acquired.

Over a hundred tea-making herbs have been mentioned in this book and thirty are illustrated. Their uses have been described and although it may sound strange, some are not for drinking!

Herbal infusions, used externally as poultices, foments, skin-tonics, eye-washes, baths, dressings for wounds and compresses, often have no equal, so some of these have been included too.

It is best, if possible, to gather your own herbs, and they can then be used fresh, or dried in an airy sheltered place, before being placed into screw-topped jars. Some, like Sage, Mint, Parsley and Borage flowers, may be gathered, put into polythene bags or other containers and kept in the freezer.

Town-dwellers who have to buy most of their herbs already prepared should explore the possibility of growing a few in tubs or window-boxes, but everyone would be wise to keep professionally prepared tinctures of a few herbs like Witch Hazel, Arnica and St John's Wort ready to hand on their first-aid shelves.

Finally, do be a little adventurous in your use of herbal teas! The days are past when anyone who openly said that they preferred to drink Chamomile, Lime flower, Rose-hip or Jasmine teas was looked at askance. It is now regarded as part of the contemporary scene that people are anxious to try out different drinks which may be on offer at vegetarian restaurants.

When trying herbal teas at home, start with small quantities and always be careful to read the directions on the packets of any you may buy. A wineglassful, or even a tablespoonful at a time may be enough of some herbal infusions, even though others can be drunk by the half-pint harmlessly.

Where there could be any doubt about the proper name of a herb that is usually known by a country name, the Latin names have been included in brackets, and the names of the tea-making herbs have been set in heavy type. If unavailable elsewhere, all the herbs can usually be obtained from health shops.

Where no specific directions are given for making a tea, *tisane* or infusion of herbs, the usual method is to pour half a pint of boiling water onto one teaspoonful (or as near as possible) of the herb and then to let it stand for a minute or two before straining.

CHAPTER ONE

HERBAL TEAS FOR SHEER DELIGHT

Tastes vary, fortunately, so that what delights some palates, may not even appeal to others. It seems impossible to believe that there is anyone who does not find pleasure in sipping **Jasmine** flower tea at times. It may, like most of the other teas, have therapeutic virtues apart from being refreshing, relieving thirst and giving pleasure, but as it comes from China, these are difficult to discover.

There do not seem to be any other reasons for

Orange flowers and buds
(*Citrus aurantium*)

Rose-hips
(*Rosa* sp.)

drinking **Rose Geranium** tea either, but an
infusion of **Red Rose** petals has some cordial
properties and **Rose-hip** tea, sweetened with clear
honey, provides the system with vitamin C.

Tilleul made from flowers of the **Lime** tree (*Tilia
europaea*), (which must be picked and dried as soon
as they start coming out in high summer when
they contain all the enticements that the tree can
produce to attract bees to pollinate them) has
many different virtues, although tea made from
older fading flowers is said to have narcotic
qualities. **Orange** flower-bud tea is often helpful
to those who find it hard to get off to sleep. It is not
always easy to obtain but can usually be found in
the larger health shops.

The more flavours that are tried in the form of

fragrant herbal teas or *tisanes*, the more discerning the palate becomes. Some are exceedingly subtle. Some are so mild that smokers can taste nothing at all, but others, like **Aniseed, Caraway** and **Dill**, which is one of the ingredients for babies' gripe water, have stronger flavours. These digestive teas come from annual aromatic herbs, natives of hotter countries, but they can be grown in Britain in hot summers, although they do not always produce mature seed.

A map showing the countries of origin of all the herbs we use for teas, for culinary purposes and even for horticultural and picturesque purposes, would indicate that they come from all over the world.

CHAPTER TWO

ALTERATIVE TEAS
'For improving the condition
of the whole system'

There are many herbs, including common garden weeds and hedgerow plants, that have been used for generations as blood-purifiers, appetite-restorers, convalescence-accelerators, and for helping the process of nutrition. They are not quite the same as tonic herbs – those will come later – but their prolonged use can do the whole body nothing but good.

Tea, or an infusion, made from **Birch** leaves, is of inestimable value to those who feel jaded after the winter. **Birch** should be picked when the young, beautiful leaves first unfold and are full of natural vitamin C. They also contain minerals which many people need and this tea is

Blue Flag
(*Iris versicolor*)

exceptionally helpful to those who suffer from rheumatic conditions. Country-folk held it in high esteem 'for the complexion' (see page 24).

Burdock makes another safe conditioning tea, as does **Fennel** (which is said to absorb poisons in the body), and **Agrimony** (*Agrimonia eupatoria*) (see also page 49), **Centaury** (*Centaurium erythraea*), **Blackberry** leaf, **Cornsilk** (*Zea mays*), **Cleavers** (*Galium aparine*), **Elder**, and **Blue Flag** (*Iris versicolor*), which grows in swamps in America and should not be confused with the garden Iris, are all supposed to be splendid for clearing the skin, a sure sign that toxic wastes are on their way

Maté
(*Ilex paraguensis*)

out.

Some of these herbal teas take a long time to fulfil their purpose and it is no good being impatient when taking them, for their action is sure, fairly slow, deep and harmless.

Maté tea (see also page 58) substituted for all ordinary Indian or China tea can become as pleasing as either and is indeed a lot better for you. Some people are slower getting to like it than others, but it is worth persevering as it has many virtues which are enough reward in themselves. It creates a feeling of well-being as well as being a soothing drink and will, in time, give a tired, poison-laden system the chance to recuperate naturally.

Curiously enough, **Maté** tea satisfies hunger and is therefore good for slimmers or those who are trying not to eat as much as usual, for there is no need to have a biscuit or a bit of cake with a cup of **Maté**!

CHAPTER THREE

CARMINATIVE TEAS
'For comforting the stomacke'

'Comforting the stomacke', of course, includes 'dispelling wind from the belly', curing nausea and stopping hiccoughs, among a host of other minor irritations.

Many of the carminative herbs are the aromatic

Angelica
(*Angelica archangelica*)

annuals (already mentioned on page 15), which are delicious in flavour even though they are tender in British gardens. This means, of course, that they must not be planted until all threat of frosts are past. During sunny summers, however, it is possible to grow a supply of seeds for kitchen use and for making herbal drinks and to keep for chewing.

Caraway, Dill, Fennel and **Anise** seeds can all be used as harmless minute snack-sweets and carried for that purpose to allay acute hunger or even boredom, as they were in the eighteenth and nineteenth centuries. They were known as 'Go to meeting seeds' then and the atmosphere in church and chapel when the sermons were too long must have become redolent with their spicy fragrance.

The **Mints**, which are hardy perennials, all make good, fast-working carminative drinks, the only dubious one, for women at least, being **Pennyroyal** which, when taken too frequently, can bring on menstruation. **Mint** greatly enhances the flavour of homemade drinks like lemonade.

Most of these aromatic herbs have been used in the distillation of liqueurs for a very long time. As they all act as digestives, it may be that this was the original purpose of these concentrated alcoholic drinks, especially at the end of the enormous rich feasts and banquets that, for example, the Romans indulged in. It is said that wedding-cake started as little spicy cakes in Roman times when they were eaten 'to alleviate over-fullness'.

In the Middle Ages when even more meat was eaten than it is now, often too regardless of its condition or age, **Cumin** was thought to be the strongest flavourer among these tasty herbs and

Sweet Cicely
(*Myrrhis odorata*)

was justly valued. **Dill**, too, played its part and
has other medicinal properties (see page 15), and
fresh leaves from the growing plant are very
pleasing in salads if they are used carefully. **Dill**
tea makes a good digestion promoting drink and it
is interesting to read that these herbs were of such
great value that they were recognized in New
Testament days as tithes.

Chamomile tea is recommended to get rid of an
unpleasant taste in the mouth and for heartburn
and colic. The plant is of great use to herbalists for
a wide variety of purposes and can safely be used
in the home without a prescription.

Lemon Balm tea was suggested by the London
Dispensary in the seventeenth century to be
'drunk every morning to renew youth, strengthen

the brain, relieve languishing nature and prevent baldness'. It is also a 'cheering' herb.

Angelica tea (*which must not be used by diabetics*, as it may cause an excess or increase of sugar in the urine) has many carminative virtues as well as being said to destroy the desire for alcohol.

An infusion of **Sweet Cicely**, a big, handsome perennial umbelliferous plant which grows wild in the north of Britain more often than the south (but which can easily be cultivated in southern counties), is a soothing digestive drink and is a gentle stimulant for debilitated stomachs.

The plant has synergic ability which means that the sweet and pleasant flavouring from its leaves combines with the acidity of sour fruits, or rhubarb, to make them taste less acid and to need less sugar, when they are cooked together.

CHAPTER FOUR

TEAS FROM CORDIAL HERBS
'To cheer the heart and spirits'

Depression is nothing new, for the cordial herbs were frequently mentioned by the old herbalists and had the reputation of being invaluable to those that were in need of 'the heart being cheereth'.

They did, in many cases, act as mild heart tonics, and so should not be used indiscriminately for teas or *tisanes*. In some cases, they should only be taken with the approval of your doctor or qualified medical herbalist.

Some of the most famous heart herbs are still in medical use, like Foxglove which is under strict prescription and must only be taken in very small

Borage
(*Borago officinalis*)

doses at any time. But there are other herbs that
are non-poisonous and contain no narcotics, like
the long fine styles that persist on each of the seeds
of **Maize**, or **Indian Corn**, to make a tassel of
Cornsilk. Tea from **Cornsilk** makes a wonderful
drink for those 'with low spirits' as well as for
several other purposes, as will be seen later in this
book.

Woodruff and **Hawthorn** are also useful
cordial herbs and some of the old herbalists used
to suggest that any of the sweet and highly-scented
flowers would have a cheering, stimulating effect
on the whole body if they were seethed, a few at a
time, in boiling water to make a fragrant tea.
Clove Pinks, Red Rose petals, **Violets, Lilies of**

the Valley, which also help the sleepless (see page 53), were often included among the cordial herbs.

Thyme tea, taken only occasionally, was said to encourage bravery and activity and 'to take away anguish'. **Lemon Balm**, with its heart-shaped leaves, made a herbal tea that John Evelyn, the diarist, said was 'sovereign for the brain', and for 'strengthening the memory and powerfully chasing away melancholy'. It was therefore said to revive the heart, and the Victorians sometimes used it to prevent young ladies from swooning at the feet of their lovers when, presumably, they were stammering out their hitherto undeclared and possibly unsuspected passions.

Borage, scentless until the young leaves are crushed, when they smell faintly of cucumber, but with the most beautiful star-shaped cobalt flowers, is the best-known cheering, cordial herb of all, providing, as Bacon said, 'a sovereign drink for melancholy passion'. It has, incidentally, a quick action, and for some people a cup of **Borage** tea lifts a slight state of depression like magic and nearly as fast.

CHAPTER FIVE

COSMETIC TEAS
'For helping to beautify the skin'

Many herbs, including most of the alterative herbs, will in time have a clearing effect on the complexion, as well as on the whole system, if drunk regularly. But there are special skin-beautifiers mentioned by the ancients, like tea made from the pale blue **Chicory** flowers which was said to 'give the plainest maid a measure of loveliness by her bright shining skin'.

Chicory got this reputation because there was
once a beautiful woman who the Sun himself
wished to marry. But she spurned him and after
she had refused he turned her into a wild Chicory
plant and ensured that her fragile flowers would
forever turn towards him, wherever he was in the
sky, from dawn until dusk. No one knows whether
this legend arose before **Chicory** had earned its
name as a complexion improving drink, or after!
But the flowers used for making a tea to drink do
seem eventually to give the skin a healthy glow.

Tea made from **Birch** leaves, if taken three
times a day for a month or more, should cure a
spotty skin, and it is claimed that **Cleavers** tea
will clear the stubbornest cases of acne in time.

Cleavers
(*Galium aparine*)

Lime flowers
(*Tilia europaea*)

AR

Chickweed picked fresh and infused in the usual way, has, it seems, been drunk in gallons over the centuries to give 'milkmaids and others' perfect complexions. Doubtless its vitamin-content was beneficial. **Scurvy-grass** (*Cochlearia officinalis*) tea is another anti-scorbutic which was thought to 'do away with all complexion blemishes', and **Hyssop** makes another skin-refresher.

All the above infusions are for internal use and should be taken a wineglassful at a time. Now for external use. Herbal teas used as appliable lotions have been in constant use by country people for hundreds and hundreds of years. There are still plenty of available plants for 'removing sandy spots vulgarly known as freckles, scattered over the face'.

The whole **Fumitory** plant was seethed to 'bathe the face night and morning', and **Darnel** (*Lolium temulentum*), known only as a rare and poisonous invading grass nowadays, used to be used to 'make the skin white and soft'. **Elder**, which is of course the herbalists' answer to so many problems, both internal and external, also took away freckles if you 'wash yr face in the wane of the moone, with a sponge, morning and evening … letting the same dry into the skin. Your water must be distilled in May', which means while the **Elder** flowers are out, according to a seventeenth-century writer.

Tea, or *tilleul*, made from **Lime** flowers was a very famous skin wash, often used in France for bathing babies. 'The Good Housewife's Handmaid' of 1585 said that a quart of **Wild Strawberries**' and **Tansy** should be infused in '3 pintes of new milke' for washing 'your face therein'. **Tansy** as a complexion lotion had many advocates (it is also a 'bitter' herb, good for the liver). Chapped hands soaked in a tea made from fresh **Groundsel** can still be made much smoother and **Blue Flag** (*Iris versicolor*) as well as the garden plant German Iris (*I. germanica*) provide similar emollient qualities.

A solution of **Eyebright** makes an invaluable eye-wash (if the tincture is used, it should be diluted with at least an equal quantity of water) and is cooling to inflamed eyes, especially, as the old herbalists used to say, 'if they look bloody'.

There is nothing so good as **Mint** tea to dab on irritating membranes including the area of the vulva when pruritus becomes unbearable. **Nettle** tea, made as usual with an ounce of the fresh herb (picked with gloves on) to a quart of boiling water, can make a harmless and very soothing cure for an itching skin due to nettle-rash. Many people find it far more efficacious than any other dabbing lotion.

It is interesting to know that the heat, burning and irritation from nettle stings themselves can be alleviated by using **Nettle** tea on them, and to realize that the actual glandular hairs on the plant that cause the stings contain a substance that is comparable with histamine. This is a good example of 'like curing like'.

In Elizabeth I's day both **Chamomile** and **Rosemary** teas were used as rinses for the hair, the former to make it as 'fair as flax' and the latter 'to burnish the hair of those that are dark'.

CHAPTER SIX

PAIN-KILLING TEAS
'For allaying the agony'

Pain-killing teas could do with a book to themselves for there are so many of them. Most of them, of course, have a variety of other therapeutic uses as well. **St John's Wort** (*Hypericum perforatum*), for example, when used as an external lotion by anyone who is unlucky enough to have their toes stamped on or their fingers crushed in a door, takes the pain away very fast.

Nettle tea makes an equally quick pain-killer when applied to burns on lint or a pad of gauze and for sunburn, and a drink of **Feverfew** (*Tanacetum parthenium*) can help to cure migraine. It used actually to be called the Headache Plant.

Carl Linnaeus, the father of modern botany,

discovered that **Wild Strawberries** cured his migraine, and other sufferers claim that **Strawberry** or **Blackberry-leaf** teas have the same value for them. Unfortunately migraine has many causes, many of them still unknown, so it is impossible to suggest a specific herbal tea to alleviate it.

Hops infused in boiling water help to lift a hangover-headache. So if the pain the next morning was caused by too much beer the night

Four pain-killing herbs for external lotions

St John's Wort
(*Hypericum perforatum*)

Nettle
(*Urtica dioica*)

Marigold
(*Calendula officinalis*)

Arnica
(*Arnica montana*)

before, it could be said that the cure lies in taking a hair of the dog that bit you!

Dandelion tea can produce good results for sufferers from bilious headaches and for those who have gall-bladder pain.

For external use once more, a dressing made from diluted **Witch Hazel** tincture, used cold, will take off the immediate agony of knocking a varicose vein, while a cloth soaked in **Comfrey** (*Symphytum officinale*) solution wrapped round a sprain or bad bruise, or even laid lightly over a simple fracture on the way to hospital, does help to quieten the pain.

Arnica will do the same in many of these cases but must never be used if there is any break in the skin.

Longer-term pain-alleviating drinks can be made from a wide variety of herbs. **Greater Celandine** (*Chelidonium majus*), which should only be prescribed by a medical herbalist, is said to help those who suffer from rheumatism of the hips and thighs, and a mixed tea made from **Agrimony** and **Dandelion** is suggested for arthritics.

Plantain tea, as hot as can be borne, held in the mouth of 'those tortured by toothacke' works wonders for some people, while **Chamomile** tea, sipped hot while resting, soon relieves colicky pains, especially those caused by wind round the navel.

Lesser Celandine or 'Pilewort' (*Ranunculus ficaria*) and **Witch Hazel** can both be used for external applications on painful piles and will often bring rapid alleviation.

CHAPTER SEVEN

ANTISEPTIC TEAS
'For cleansing purposes'

There are medical herbalists, especially in America and Europe, who now claim antibiotic properties for some herbs. **Nasturtium** (*Tropaeolum majus*), they say, can be used in some cases instead of more orthodox antibiotics, as can **Garden Cress** (*Lepidium sativum*) and **Mouse-eared Hawkbit** (*Hieracium pilosella*).

    Round-leaved Sundew (*Drosera rotundifolia*) which has long been advocated as a herbal and a homoeopathic cure for acute barking coughs like

Fennel
(*Foeniculum vulgare*)

whooping cough, is, they say, another antibiotic herb, together with one or two lichens.

It is essential, of course, that these herbs for bacteria-killing purposes must be prescribed medically but anyone can eat **Nasturtium** leaves in salads, or make soup (as a form of herbal tea) from **Watercress** (*Nasturtium officinale*) as long as they get it from an unpolluted source.

But to go on to antiseptic, as opposed to anti-biotic, herbs (antiseptic in this case being taken to mean that these herbs contain a substance which arrests or prevents putrefaction), perhaps **Meadowsweet** is the best known, or one of them, for internal use. This delightful plant, which used to be so common in Britain, gets scarcer whenever man drains the fields in which it used to grow, but if some can be obtained, it is a useful herb to keep (and easy to dry) for making teas all the year round. It is good for digestive troubles, inflammation of the urinary system, or for feverish colds, and was one of the three most sacred herbs of the Druids.

The **Mints** and other old garden herbs, **Marjoram, Sage, Hyssop, Fennel** and **Thyme**, all have antiseptic virtues, which may be one of the reasons why they have always been so popular for culinary and medical purposes.

As an antiseptic external poultice herb there is nothing to touch an infusion of **St John's Wort**. Countless cures of septic wounds are recited by herbalists in praise of this herb as well as the efficacy in preventing lockjaw from dirty wounds and accidents in the garden. A woman was saying only the other day how her husband ran one of the tines of a fork right through his boot, straight into his foot. She poured a solution of **St John's Wort** straight into the wound and it healed quickly and without any other treatment.

It is just as good for scratches from pets' claws, stab-wounds from splinters and thorns, and any cuts which may have become infected, all of which are common happenings in family life.

An interesting side-line about all these antiseptic herbs is that in the old days, before carpets were in general use, everyone used what were known as **Strewing herbs** as floor coverings. **Meadowsweet**, all the **Mints, Marjoram** and **Thyme** were in demand for this purpose, and others ostensibly more fragrant like Sweet Flags and Sweet Woodruff which were often used 'for my lady's chamber', not only for their sweet smell but for their antiseptic virtues too.

CHAPTER EIGHT

DIAPHORETIC TEAS
'For provoking a sweat'

The names of some herbs, as will have been noticed already in this book, occur over and over again in herbal treatments. They may appear in different contexts altogether as being of use in a wide variety of out-of-health situations.

One of these particularly useful herbs is gathered very easily in high summer from the low branches of the **Lime** tree (*Tilia europaea*), for **Lime** flowers, as well as being of great help 'to those who are wakeful' when taken as a bed-time *tisane* and those who seek a pleasing drink at all times, are good too for those who feel hot and bothered at the start of a cold. In such cases **Lime** flower tea provokes a gentle sweat which may be

in time to knock the incipient cold on the head, as
it were.

There is **Marjoram** too, a plant that grows
on the chalk hills in Britain, which is highly
aromatic in all its parts, leaves, stems, roots, and
the purple flowers that are so sought out by bees
and the little blue butterflies which inhabit these
hills. **Marjoram** tea has many uses, among them
its ability to start off a stimulation of the sweat
glands, or taken in small quantities, to help to
change a taut, over-dry skin in such unpleasant
illnesses as influenza to a satisfactorily supple,
moist state again.

Tea made from **Thyme, Marjoram's**
neighbour on the hills, is also suggested as a

Yarrow
(*Achillea millefolium*)

diaphoretic drink as well as that from the invasive **Lemon Balm**, a member of the same botanic tribe, which grows like a rampageous weed in some gardens.

Two common roadside weeds, **Burdock** and **Yarrow** are recommended by some herbalists as sweat-provokers. **Burdock**, which is sometimes called 'Sweethearts' because of its seeds' hooked tips which are loath to let passers-by through narrow gaps without clinging to them, is a good general health tea as well as being diaphoretic. **Yarrow**, 'of a million leaves' as well as of a million uses, may be the most famous of the sweat-encouragers but it should always be used with care or its action may be too drastic.

Viper's Bugloss, with rough leaves and stems but spires of handsome blue flowers, is highly thought of by some herbalists for the same purpose.

But perhaps it is the dual co-operation of **Elder** and **Peppermint**, making a tea to be sipped while very hot with the addition of a squeeze of lemon and honey, that provides the best-known 'sweat-exciter' of all. Certainly both **Elder** and **Peppermint** have many other attributes too, but this does not make them any less useful in this particular case.

CHAPTER NINE

DIURETIC TEAS
'For promoting the urine'

Those who have ever suffered any difficulty in passing urine, or from cystitis (the name that covers a variety of symptoms of inflammation of

Couch Grass
(*Agropyron repens*)

the urinary system) or the pain of prostate troubles, should be prepared to understand the importance of the diuretic herbs.

As the causes of the inflammation always vary a great deal, it is often difficult to know immediately which of these herbal teas will be of most help. But give one a good chance, especially if it has been carefully prescribed for your condition, before moving on to try another.

Many herbs have been found, over the years, to be useful in relieving both the tension set up by sheer soreness of passing over-acid urine and in helping to change the acidity to a less irritating and burning alkalinity, and also to have a basic value in lessening the inflammation and sometimes the obstructions that produce so much pain. It is essential to consult a medical herbalist but it is interesting, too, to know something about these helpful herbs.

A tea made from **Cleavers** (*Galium aparine*), one of the commonest weeds in garden and countryside and sometimes called 'Little Sweethearts' in the country (see page 34, **Burdock**), makes a mild diuretic tea which is of great value in many cases. It can be drunk half a pint at a time and may not taste of anything much except 'greenery', but it is suggested for those 'with a sudden chill in the bladder after standing on cold ground and being smitten upwards'. It is also recommended for burning pains in the urethra.

Celery seed tea, **Marsh Mallow** tea (for its

Marsh Mallow
(*Althaea officinalis*)

very mucilaginousness and soothing ability – this is a demulcent tea), **Couch Grass** 'water' (see page 39) and infusions of **Dandelion**, or **Parsley Piert** (*Aphanes arvensis*) serve the purpose of increasing the flow of urine. The hard leaves of **Bearberry,** (*Arctostaphylos uva ursi*) and those of a South African plant **Buchu** (*Barosma betulina*) suit some people well, but the pride of place goes to two American herbs, or herbs that originally came from the States; one of these is **Cornsilk**, the tassels that sprout off the tips of **Maize** seeds on the cob, and the other is **Gravelroot**, or Purple Boneset (*Eupatorium purpuratum*). **Cornsilk** tea can work very fast as a general soothing herb and diuretic, and quickly alleviates much bladder soreness and urethral pain. It is harmless and quarter-pint doses can be repeated frequently. **Gravelroot** tea is often very helpful to prostate sufferers as well as others needing a safe diuretic tea. This herb is also known as 'Joe Pye', or 'Trumpetweed'.

Herbalists recommend **Pipsissewa** tea for helping a dropsical state caused by water retention, as well as for urinary discomfort. The common name comes straight from the Indians, from whom the whole world has learnt of so many of our best herbal remedies. **Pipsissewa** is instantly onomatopoeic of someone getting rid of their urine at a good healthy rate! It is made from the evergreen plant of *Chimophila umbellata*.

Butcher's Broom, or 'Knee Holly', one of the British woodland, prickly, evergreen features of the winter countryside, was also used as a diuretic and some modern herbalists still suggest a course of tea made from it. Culpeper thought highly of it, saying that a 'Decoction of the root made with wine openeth obstructions, provoketh urine and helpeth to expel gravel and the stone'. It is just as good as a herbal tea made with water, for wine often only inflames already sore urinary organs.

Perhaps it is interesting to mention that many of the herbs used for making diuretic teas have, as they get rid of surplus water in the system, a slimming effect on some people. They should not, however, be used haphazardly for this purpose without consulting a medical herbalist, with the exception, perhaps, of **Cleavers** which makes a harmless slimming tea.

CHAPTER TEN

TEAS TO HELP COUGHS AND COLDS

As may be guessed, tradition, culled from an accumulation of knowledge from ancient to modern times, plus news of miracle medicines which travellers from all over the world have brought in, has led to a multitude of suggested herbal teas for helping those with coughs and colds.

The diaphoretic herbs, if used directly a cold is suspected, particularly in the evening before going to bed, will often dispel it altogether.

But once a cold in the head has got a grip on the system all that can be done is to try to control it in the least annoying manner.

Sage, which was originally brought to Britain by the Romans, possibly to disguise the flavour of coarse or rancid meats, or even to bring out flavours of tasteless foods, as well as for medicinally useful purposes, makes an excellently

Elder
(*Sambucus nigra*)

soothing gargle. During the history of its use by man, **Sage** has earned itself the reputation of having many virtues, including the propensity for giving long life, and was recommended for anyone 'that hath no speech in sickness' when one should 'take the juice of sage and put it in the patient's mouth when by the grace of God, it shall make him speak'.

Couch Grass tea (*Agropyrum repens*), which has other uses, can be helpful in the early stages of catarrhal troubles.

Oswego Tea (see Introduction) made from the young leaves of the **Crimson Bergamot** (*Monarda didyma*) which, like others in the Mint tribe, contain thymol, an antiseptic oil or indeed **Thyme** itself, which is infused for colds in hot milk in some

European countries – will sometimes lessen the unpleasantness of bronchial troubles if taken soon and regularly enough.

But once colds are in full swing, many herbalists recommend 'Composition Essence' diluted in water. This remedy contains both famous herbs **Elder** and **Peppermint** again. Composition Essence can be obtained from most health shops.

Cornsilk tea is useful in obstinate cases of catarrh, as is an infusion of **Borage**. Both are demulcent, somewhat mucilaginous herbs, so are further examples of the old precept of 'like curing like'.

There are people who swear by **Fennel** tea for colds, others rely on a decoction of **Yarrow** or on the very well-known even if old-fashioned in this

Mint
(*Mentha piperita*)

day and age, remedy of **Coltsfoot**. Its virtues were often extolled in the Middle Ages because it was such a common plant, the idea being that the more common a plant or weed was, the greater its value, or perhaps, the more uses it could be put to.

Smokers with sore chests would do well to try tobacco made from dried **Coltsfoot** leaves instead of ordinary and possibly adulterated 'mixtures'.

Camphor and Cinnamon from the Far East are among the most valuable of all the herbs for colds and bronchial troubles, and diluted tincture of Squills (*Urginea scilla*) and Balsam tolu (*Myroxylon toluifera*), often used in cough lozenges, still have their uses. But all these have to be imported and herbs growing nearer home can serve the same purposes.

Plenty of hedgerow herbs, like **Horehound** (*Marrubium vulgare*) and even, so it is said, **Duckweed** (*Lemna minor*), as well as the handsome **Elecampane** (*Inula helenium*) which flourishes in some damp meadows in Britain, all make good teas for coughs and colds. In fact, the last named has the reputation with some herbalists for being a specific herb to help stubborn, tickling coughs finally to vanish.

CHAPTER ELEVEN

FEBRIFUGE TEAS
'To allay the fever'

Feverfew, the magic herb for some migraine sufferers, comes, strictly speaking, into the category of a fever-reducing herb. Indeed, the herbalist Eleanour Sinclair Rohde, who wrote many enchanting books earlier this century, went as far as to say that it was used as our forefathers' aspirin (and a good deal less harmful it was too) and was also though to be good for reducing blood-pressure.

How interesting it will be when pharmacognosists and physicians put their knowledge together even more deeply and generally than is now being done, to find out the exact action the various elements in herbs have on

Feverfew
(*Tanacetum parthenium*)

Centaury
(*Centaurium erythraea*)

different parts of the body; also, perhaps, why and when and how they have different effects on different people and at different times of their lives.

Meanwhile, however, we go on chiefly by tradition and the accumulated reputations of plant virtues which have been derived empirically through the centuries. But as science delves deeper and deeper into the properties of herbal medicine, it is satisfactory to many who have always relied on it to hear that these old uses have a basis in physical fact.

Tea from **Borage** leaves, as well as warm and short drinks of an infusion of **Hyssop** can both be helpful in reducing fevers. A small, pink-flowered wild plant, **Centaury** (*Centaurium erythraea*), makes another febrifuge tea but not one that should be taken unless prescribed by a qualified herbalist, although in Devonshire it is known as 'Feverwort' and has obviously been in frequent country use there in the past. It has, too, the curious reputation for killing lice, but whether it discourages these body vermin to leave their hosts when it is imbibed as a drink, or whether the use has to be by external dabbing, is not described. Tea from **Centaury** and **Agrimony** together used to be given as a remedy 'against the Ague or Malaria'.

Both **Yarrow** and **Hyssop** teas were often used to reduce the temperature with a wonderful variety of other herbs and ingredients. The recipe of a seventeenth-century concoction known as 'The Water of Life', only to be given, not surprisingly, 'a few drops at a time for fevers' as well as in health 'as a strengthening tonic', is so interesting that it is quoted in full from an old herb book. To make 'The Water of Life' it was necessary to:

Take Balm leaves and stalks, Betony leaves and flowers, Rosemary, Red Sage, Taragon, Tormentil leaves, Rossolis and Roses, Carnation, Hyssop, Thyme, red strings that grow upon Savory, red Fennel leaves and root, red Mints, of each a handful; bruise these hearbes and put them in a great earthen pot and pour on them enough White Wine as will cover them, stop them close, and let them steep for eight or nine days; then put to it Cinnamon, Ginger, Angelica-seeds, Cloves and Nuttmegs, of each an ounce, a little Saffron, Sugar one pound, Raysins solis stoned one pound, Dates stoned and sliced half a pound, the loyns and legs of an old Coney [rabbit], a fleshy running Capon, the red flesh of the sinews of a leg of Mutton, four young Chickens, twelve Larks, the yolks of twelve eggs, a Loaf of White Bread, cut in sops; and two or three ounces of Mithridate or Treacle, and as much Muscadine as will cover them all.

The mixture had to be distilled at 'a moderate fire'.

CHAPTER TWELVE

TEAS FOR FOMENTS AND COMPRESSES
'For drawing out the bad'

Many herbal infusions used to be used externally for stimulating areas of the skin, or indeed for heating them up, as well as for increasing the circulation or dilating the blood vessels of the part to which they were applied.

These foments are still of great value for the above purposes as well as for soothing the endings of the nerves on or near the skin, so they both help the absorption of effusions and relieve pain. They can also be used to soften the skin when there are boils, abscesses and carbuncles, and to 'bring these localized inflammations up or to draw them to a point'.

For the last purpose a tiny plant which often grows on old walls and is still known as **Whitlow-grass** (*Erophila verna*) was said to be incomparable, while **Marsh Mallow** (*Althaea officinalis*), still in common use by modern herbalists, ought to be known far more widely. This wild plant grows near the sea, and has large velvety leaves which, when steeped in boiling water, produce an excellent 'drawing' solution applied while still hot to help to ripen and draw all boils, abscesses and carbuncles.

Plantain
(*Plantago major*)

Plantain tea is said to help unreachable tooth-abscesses if held hot in the mouth.

An old-fashioned, cruel, blistering foment which has now been virtually dispensed with, but which deserves a mention to show differences in modern attitudes, was made from a very strong **Capsicum** infusion, with the addition of Cantharides, which was used on people as well as animals in order to cause a counter-irritant to lameness and other inflammations by raising blisters on the skin. The only useful relic of this performance nowadays is the use of **Capsicum**-treated cotton-wool as *dry* 'chest-warmers', 'sore-joint-protectors' or abdominal belts.

Instead of blistering as a means to achieving the eventual cure of deeper sources of pain, it is more helpful to try, say, an infusion of **Marjoram** on a thick pad of lint, put on as hot as the flesh can bear to soothe localized rheumaticky pains. These foments, frequently used by people living in villages among chalk downland within living memory, were said to be 'better than anything else for the screws'. **Marjoram** has the additional virtue of 'curing those who are much given to sighing'!

As boils, abscesses or carbuncles start healing, a foment made from **Cleavers** tea is said to help to produce a healthy granulation of flesh instead of too abundant a production of proudflesh.

Figwort (*Scrophularia nodosa*), a common brown-

Lavender
(*Lavendula vera*)

flowered plant, much favoured by visiting wasps, provides a useful herb from which to make a foment for curing the swelling of sprains. So, of course, does the Accident Plant, or **Arnica**, but this only grows in mountainous countries and is usually sold in tincture form. The young leaves of **Comfrey** (*Symphytum officinale*), made into an infusion and applied cold on a cloth, take away the sharp pain of bruises direct on to bones like the shin. Actually, **Comfrey** is a useful herb in all cases of bone injury.

On a large scale, herbal teas made from different aromatic herbs greatly improve and provide helpful additions to bath-water. There is nothing as refreshing as a **Rosemary** or a **Pine** bath, and for either of these about a quarter of a pound of branch-tips should be cut and infused for half an hour, or even boiled for a few minutes, in a quart of water. The resulting green tea can be strained and poured straight into the bath just before it is used. *Do not use* **Rosemary**, or **Pine** at night as they are both stimulating and may prevent you from going to sleep, but a **Lavender** bath, made in the same way, if there is enough of the plant to spare, is soothing before sleep.

CHAPTER THIRTEEN

TEAS FOR 'TAKING AWAY BILIOUSNESS'

It sounds rather as if our forefathers often suffered from bouts of liverishness, for there are countless references to herbs for 'drawing out the bile' or to those for 'helping them with naughty livers'. Primarily, it was to the bitter herbs that they fled every time – the herbs used traditionally at the Feast of the Passover, all of which are beneficial for mild liver complaints, like **Mugwort, Tansy, Horehound, Agrimony** (see page 16), and particularly any part of **Dandelion**. All were helpful in getting rid of the effects of over-indulgence which might have caused 'the lethargy'.

Dandelion tea, made in the usual way with an ounce of fresh herb to a pint of boiling water, not only counteracts biliousness but acts as a mild diuretic and slimming herb and is, internally this time, 'helpful to them who suffer from the screws', the name so graphically given by country-workers to rheumaticky pain. It also makes a mild laxative

Dandelion
(*Taraxacum officinale*)

drink and provides a bevy of mineral salts including calcium, iron, magnesium, potassium and silicon for the system as well.

Nothing could be more easy to find than **Dandelions** and as all parts of the plant can be used and there is no need to wait for the flowers or buds, it is nearly always available. It is surprisingly helpful for those who never feel 'quite up to scratch' and well worth trying for a month or two.

Greater Celandine (*Chelidonium majus*) is another famous 'liver' herb. It is nothing like its junior namesake, **Lesser Celandine**, or Pilewort, to look at, except that both have yellow flowers. **Greater Celandine** is a bigger plant and is a member of the same botanical family as the poppy. It has a yellow milky juice which shows up as soon as any part of the plant is bruised or broken and it

Barberry
(*Berberis vulgaris*)

was this, it seems, which first led the old herbalists to suppose that, as this juice looked the colour of bile, it should be good to help liver upsets. It is an example of the 'Doctrine of Signatures', (see the Introduction to *Herbs For First-aid and Minor Ailments*, Everybody's Home Herbal Series, Thorsons Publishers Ltd.)

The old plant-gatherers and users were perfectly correct and *Chelidonium*, or **Greater Celandine**, is still used by modern herbalists. However it is not a plant for the amateur to try and must be prescribed by a medical herbalist.

Yarrow, Broom, Bogbean (*Menyanthes trifoliata*), **Barberry**, and **Centaury** teas may all be prescribed for bilious conditions and some of these herbs may be compounded for use by skilled practitioners, but for home, self-use, **Dandelion** tea is the safest standby for helping liverishness.

CHAPTER FOURTEEN

TEAS TO INDUCE SLEEP
'And help to settle obstreporous spirits'

The list of harmless herbs to help the nerves, to get people through periods of stress and to induce healthy sleep is so long that it is surprising that anyone has to take to harmful, habit-forming tranquillizers and sleeping-pills.

The familiar herb **Chamomile** (see page 20) comes at the top perhaps, closely followed by **Hops** 'for unstrung conditions of the nervous system' and the aforementioned **Lime** flowers, which feature so often in this book.

Tea made from **Oats** is good as well, and of

course tradition has it that it is oatmeal which has been responsible for making the Scots into such a fine strong race. **Oat** tea is especially helpful if as well as a strung-up state, there is a perpetual headache, niggling away all the time. It also makes a good bedtime drink for those who 'fidget after sleep' as well as for those who are suffering from nervous exhaustion.

Perhaps **Skullcap** (*Scutellaria lateritiflora*) sometimes spelled Scullcap, is the best known of the sedative herbs and a tea made from this plant, which is not a native of Britain, is soothing to the nerves and particularly helps those who suffer

Oats
(*Avena sativa*)

Passion-flower
(*Passiflora incarnata*)

from twitchiness and general restlessness.
Valerian (*Valeriana offinalis*) has an ancient
reputation but must only be taken on prescription
because it is dangerous to mix it with orthodox
medical drugs. It is often helpful for over-sensitive
people and for those who, once off to sleep at
night, feel that they are floating in the air!
Valerian tea will also help those who are
extremely irritable, or who frequently have
pressure in their foreheads, or an outstandingly
cold head. As a sideline, it also helps people who
start choking or coughing a lot directly they start
falling asleep.

  Wild Lettuce tea, **Orange** flower-bud tea, **Lily
of the Valley** tea, **Cowslip** tea and even such
exotic herbal teas as that made from **Passion-**

flowers (*Passiflora incarnata*) are all helpful to those who have to woo sleep and then fail to catch it!

Herbalists may suggest a course of **Yellow Moccasin Flower** (*Cypripedium pubescens*) tea for soothing purposes. It was introduced, or so it is said, into the official American Materia Medica by Professor Rafinesque who was once Professor of Medical Botany at the University of Transylvania. It had obviously been a traditional Indian herbal medicine, but Professor Rafinesque is thought to have proved its efficacy more recently and found that the flowers produce beneficial results in all nervous diseases and hysterical states without any baneful or harmful or narcotic effects.

Valerian
(*Valeriana officinalis*)

After such an exotic plant it is pleasing to be able to come back to one of our homeliest and most common garden herbs, mentioned often before, for **Sage** makes a nerve-soothing tea and can be drunk without any worry of side-effects. If you treat yourself it is always wiser to mention the fact to your doctor or herbalist, in case any of the herbs do not 'marry with' any others that qualified herbalists may prescribe for you.

CHAPTER FIFTEEN

TEAS FOR TONICS
'For improving the tone and vigour of the system'

In the old days before vegetables were cultivated much in gardens, our ancestors probably missed the benefits we now gain from having fresh 'greens' available all the year round. It would appear that after long, cold, 'shut-in' winters they usually took to dosing themselves with spring tonics in the form of **Nettle** tea (which they also frequently fermented to produce **Nettle** beer), and all kinds of other blood-purifying herbal drinks.

Sage leaf tea came into its own yet again, especially for convalescents, as did refreshing **Birch** leaf drinks, and all the virtues ascribed to vitamin-producing **Cowslips** and **Primroses** brought them into use. Perhaps it is a relic of the past that people have so much love for seeing 'the first pale primrose' appearing each year; they may create a memory of the time when their forefathers used them for health reasons, after all the dried and salted-down foods that they had survived upon during the dark months.

Actually, it is not many years since the

Cowslip
(*Primula veris*)

homoeopathic physician, Dr Dorothy Shepherd, who practised in London, used to tell worried parents of children who would not eat cooked or raw vegetables without making a great fuss, to let them pick a few cowslips, primroses or even violet flowers and either eat them straightaway or put them into sandwiches of thin wholewheat bread and butter. She used to say that a few fresh, even if unusual, 'herbs' would make all the difference to their diet. She also suggested **Primrose** and **Cowslip** teas for them to drink, but in these days of stringent conservation and rapid scarcening of wild flowers, it would possibly be easier to let them grow their own cress or parsley and eat that.

Most children will chew fresh mint leaves, or drink green **Mint** tea. Others enjoy chewing the

'Go to meeting seeds', (see page 19) or finding **Sorrel** from which to make an excellent tonic drink. **Bistort** (*Polygonum bistortum*), which is rarer than **Sorrel**, makes one of the best spring tonic teas of all and was used sometimes at Easter to make 'Easter Puddings' as well as a vitamin-giving tea.

Maté tea, taken regularly instead of ordinary tea, has a tonic effect as well as many other beneficial attributes. It contains no tannin, which is one of the faults of our more familiar **Camellia** teas from India, Ceylon or China teas.

Birch
(*Betula pendula*)

Maté tea (see also page 17) is made from the leaves of a tree (*Ilex paraguayensis*) that once only grew in South America but has now been cultivated in other tea-growing areas. It is good for rheumatism, and is a mild aperient and a tonic for the kidneys. It is also a slimming drink and after an initial sip or two becomes pleasing to the taste. Initially, it may seem a little smoky, but some people add a slice of lemon and/or a little honey to each cup to counteract this.

Maté tea must be drunk fresh. It is no good making a pint of it, like other herbal teas, unless you are going to drink it all at one sitting, because it goes black very fast after it has been brewed.

CHAPTER SIXTEEN

TEAS FOR DRESSINGS
'To heal all manner of wounds'

In the past plants designated as cures for 'all manner of wounds' often earned the name of 'woundworts', and 'wort', the Anglo-Saxon word for 'weed', has persisted through the ages in country names for plants.

There are plenty of other herbs, however, which can still be used as external vulneraries and promote far quicker and healthier healing than the strong modern antiseptic solutions that are sold for the same purpose.

Witch Hazel is one of them and it may be the best known for applying to bruises rather than other wounds or cuts, but it is immediately soothing to thorn scratches and mild abrasions as well. **Witch Hazel** is also helpful to sore eyes if applied in solution on pads of lint which are then placed over the eyes.

A somewhat less known herb, found wild in Britain, comes a good second in the list of vulneraries and those who use it would probably place it at the top of the list. This is **St John's Wort** (*Hypericum perforatum*). It is a pain-killer (see page 27) as well as a killer of some harmful bacteria, and, as has been mentioned, many reliable herbalists have given it the credit for killing the lockjaw or Tetanus bug when it is used quickly on dirty wounds – as soon as possible, indeed, after the injury has taken place. It certainly works well and many herbally-inclined families are never without a bottleful of *Hypericum* tincture on their first-aid shelf.

St John's Wort
(*Hypericum perforatum*)

Tincture of **Marigold** is very useful indeed for
clean wounds like cuts from knives. There is
nothing that will promote faster healing and that
is why it is described as for *clean wounds only* as its
healing programme is sometimes too fast for dirty
injuries to the flesh.

Nettle tea is a specific for burns and scalds. If it
is used immediately it prevents ordinary kitchen
mishaps from blistering and takes away the pain
very fast.

The actual **Woundworts** themselves (*Stachys*
spp.) of which there are at least four in Britain
belonging to the same genus, have traditional
reputations for rapid healing. Gerard writes about
a clown who cured a wound with **Common
Woundwort** (*Stachys arvensis*) applications in a
week, which was apparently much faster than
other remedies could have done it. The old
herbalist has nothing but praise for the plant's
healing of 'grievous and mortal wounds'.

There is also a herb, rare in Britain, called
Saracen's Woundwort (*Senecio fluviatilis*), which is
thought to have been brought here by the
Crusaders originally, after they discovered it to be
a wonderful cure for their own and their horses'
wounds.

Anne Pratt mentions an entertaining tale about
Woundwort being cultivated by a Mr Holton in
the nineteenth century. He demonstrated its
possibilities as a root vegetable in times of need as
well as its vulnerary virtues, and was awarded a
silver 'Ceres' medal by the Society of Arts for his
work.

And finally **Wood Betony** (*Betonica officinalis*) is
sometimes known, in different parts of the
country, as a woundwort. More often, however, it

takes the lovely country name of 'Self heal', but to many people this already belongs to the purple flowered 'Carpenter's weed' (*Prunella vulgaris*). Country names, although charming, interesting and most picturesque at times, are not enough to know for a study, even an elementary one, of the medical properties of herbs. There are other 'self-heals' and plenty of 'all-heals' and 'heal-alls' and the only way to be certain of having the correct one at the right time is to know and recognize its scientific Latin name. English and country names, or popular names, are too ambiguous to be reliable.

THERAPEUTIC INDEX

Other books for better health the natural way.

COLOUR HEALING
Chromotherapy and How It Works
Mary Anderson

Psychologically we are all affected by colour. This book explains a revolutionary new method of healing by which the rays from coloured lamps are applied to diseased organs of the body, with amazingly beneficial results.

HOW TO EAT FOR HEALTH
Diet Reform Simplified
Stanley Lief N.D., D.O., D.C.

A sensible and logical presentation of health principles based on diet, of interest and value to both experienced diet reformer and beginner alike. Explains the amount of food to be eaten, how to construct a rational diet, what to eat and when and how to eat. Includes over seventy mouth-watering recipes.

FIRST AID NATURE'S WAY
Safe and Effective Treatments for Minor Injuries and Ailments
R. Newman Turner N.D., D.O.

This is more than just a manual of basic emergency measures; it also contains treatments to hasten recovery, including homoeopathy and massage of acupressure 'points'. In addition to accidents the book deals with boils, chilblains, eyestrain, 'flu, toothache, and other ailments.

ABOUT MOLASSES
Natural Food – Natural Remedy

Molasses, a product of the sugar cane, is rich in minerals and vitamins. This book explains the amazing therapeutic properties of molasses and provides a selection of molasses recipes.